Don't Sweat It

Control Your Sweating Naturally

Emily James

Table of Contents

Introduction

Everyone sweats. It's a natural thing. It is our body cooling itself and it is necessary. But it can be uncomfortable and embarrassing when you over-sweat. As a sufferer of hyperhidrosis (excessive sweating) myself, I know exactly how it feels to feel extra sticky and wet.

And so I have come up with many different ways to control sweating naturally. I have undergone **endoscopic thoracic sympathectomy (ETS)** to fix it, but I know that not everyone can afford such surgery, and sometimes the surgery does not work 100%.

Even for people who do not suffer from hyperhidrosis, I'm sure many of you would still love to not have to deal with sweating.

Before anything else, I would just like to say that I am not a doctor nor do I have a medical background. The advice, treatments, remedies, and guidelines I give throughout the book are only my opinions.

Please feel free to use this book as you see fit, but remember that all the information contained within these pages is just that: information.

If you feel that any of the treatments might work for you, I strongly recommend that you to consult your doctor, a trained medical professional, or a trained herbalist, or other such trained professional, before you go through with any of the them. Make sure you are not allergic to any substances that you are planning to use.

Being careful is always better than sorry. Checking with someone who is able to give you an accurate assessment of the situation is for your own benefit.

It doesn't matter whether you're reading this because you think the information contained within these pages is useful or whether you're reading this with the same covert desperation that I always felt whenever I had to face up to my sweaty problems, or if you think someone you know might need help.

What matters is that you're here and that you are reading this book. I hope that you will be able to find at least something that is useful to help you with your sweaty problems.

This is how I see the 4 different types of people:

- Those who sweat normally, who know that sweating is a natural thing and accept it

- Those who sweat normally, who know that sweating is natural but who don't accept it

- Those who sweat excessively as a result of many different factors (hyperhidrosis)

- And those who don't sweat at all, or only minimally (anihidrosis)

The first two types are the people who sweat normally and they are who most people are. The last two types, those are polar opposites: they either sweat excessively or not at all. These types are not as common and, more importantly, they herald a probable medical condition.

We sweat to cool our bodies down, and also to get rid of get rid of waste matter from our bodies. Most of the time people will sweat in "normal" levels, depending on the circumstances in which they find themselves.

There is no ruler or measurement to what "normal" constitutes, but it can be taken to be moderate sweating at appropriate times, like on a hot day, when we're doing labor intensive work, or when we're nervous or excited or any other such tension inducing emotional moment.

Nevertheless, when a person overly sweats, or when they sweat "buckets", this is viewed as excessive sweating. This is also referred to in more medical terms as Hyperhidrosis.

The opposite of this condition is the person who sweats almost little to nothing at all. This is referred to as Anihidrosis.

These two conditions are not what are considered as "normal" among the medical community. They are both generally accepted to be a result of an underlying medical condition, or due to the genetic makeup of the person.

If you fall into either one of these two categories and you have no knowledge of whether any of your relatives have the same problem, it is best to consult a physician and try to find out what the underlying condition is.

This is a good way to see if you can rule out any medical causes for your excessive sweating, or non-sweating conditions. And once you've ruled out medical causes, you can then turn to treatment methods to help you fight the battle with sweat.

Those who battle with sweat are only those of us who sweat excessively. This is not an issue for those of you who only sweat minimally or not all and you will find that your life is sweat free and just great as it is.

However, people who sweat normally sometimes don't want to sweat at all. They would prefer not to have to deal with embarrassing stains, stickiness and odors. Most would prefer if they didn't have to deal with sweat at all, on any level.

There are many different manufacturers selling different brands of deodorants and antiperspirants highlighting how carefree people are when they stay sweat free. But there's simply no way to stay totally sweat free; it is not normal. Not even undergoing endoscopic thoracic sympathectomy (ETS) will be able to do so.

ETS can also have side effects such as sympathectomy: compensatory sweating (CS) and this is unfortunately quite common with most patients experiencing it to some degree.

The whole point of my book is not to show you how to stop sweating, but to share with you methods on how to control your sweating naturally, and how to minimize your sweating using natural means.

I am not here to give you the impression that I have the key to help you to stop sweating. I am one of those people who prefer to smell shower-fresh most of the time, and so I have many viable natural methods which can be used to help you control your sweating or even minimize it.

I have tried many different products out there; most of them disappoint me and some worked to a certain level. Some of them I used continuously, some only for a few weeks and others for a few days. The one thing they all have in common is that they are natural. No chemicals - and they all worked for me on some level or other.

Some worked better than others, but I still think that these are better than using chemical laden commercial deodorants and antiperspirants. There is only one reason that I didn't stick with any of them diligently:

- My dedication. Sometimes I found drifting back towards the easier, more attainable commercial varieties.

You might ask, "then why on earth do I even bothered including them in this book to begin with?" My reason:

- Know that a method which works for one person doesn't and won't, necessarily work for another person.

  Most of the methods I mention here have been tried and tested by many people; they do work, just not for everyone.

It took many trial and errors to come up with these methods, but I now I can truly say that I no longer rely on antiperspirants to keep me feeling fresh all day long.

You might like to try a few different methods instead of just constantly using just one or two. See what works best for you and all of which are easy to do.

All That Sweat and Smell

Since this book is about seat and what you can do about it, so let's go into more detail about sweat, shall we?

Hundreds of years ago, our lives were simpler and we didn't have as many harmful substances littering the earth, nor did we use toxic substances on a daily basis on our bodies and take it as normal.

Today toxins are littering not only the earth but also our bodies. Even though this might have been acceptable past, a different trend of thought has been slowly emerging. People are paying more attention to this problem.

Now we are more careful with the things we eat, what we do and what we wear and less on the world around us. We rarely take the time to stop and smell the roses, instead we take the time to stop and smell our own selves, and if this scent is anything less than pleasing we quickly become embarrassed and convinced that everyone can smell us from a mile away.

That is hardly what's going on. Of course sometimes we could notice some strong unpleasant body odor walks by, but otherwise if someone is sweating normally and the odor is not so bad, we hardly notice it at all.

We can sometimes obsessed over our "bad" smell to an extent that sometimes we find it difficult to go out in public without any type of deodorants, antiperspirants and perfumes because we believe that we smell bad.

Most people won't notice anything unless there is something radically wrong. The problem that arises here however, is the definition of radically wrong.

Do you notice giant sweat rings under your underarms, or the dots of sweat oozing down your back? What about feeling your shoes are slippery inside because of your feet are wet from sweat?

It is not easy to switch from the readily available antiperspirants and deodorants on the market (what we are used to), to the usage of natural deodorants and antiperspirants.

You can't just snap your fingers and the change will be in an instant; it is gradual, so there can be times when you're on your quest for a great natural deodorant that you might find yourself sweating buckets when you're in public. This is without the additional complication of having hyperhidrosis.

Sometimes we give up and we go back to our chemical laden deodorants and antiperspirants to get rid of our embarrassing times of sweating unconditionally behind us.

For some people, they have a reaction to all these chemical substances you're putting on your skin, and you have no choice but to turn to natural products. That reaction is mostly likely be an allergic reaction to one or more chemicals in the product you're using.

In my case, one of the reactions I had was my underarms became very itchy from deodorants and they turned dark. The dermatologist said it could be because of the alcohol or the perfume used in the product.

It took me a lot of time, patience and energy to get me where I am today.

And although I make no promises or guarantees that you will be sweat free if you use the methods and recommendations I have mentioned in this book, I can say that if you at least give them a try, you might find yourself pleasantly surprised by the outcome.

With that said, keep in mind that none of these natural remedies work immediately. You won't get one- or two-hour results. You will need to give it at least a week or two to see results.

For best results you will have to give it at least about a month. This is how long it will take your body to adapt to the fact that you're not trying to force-feed it toxic chemicals anymore.

If you tried one thing and it doesn't work, try another method. It's as simple as that. There are many methods available to you, and you can keep experimenting with them until you find the one that works best for you. This is what I did to reach the point where I am now.

If you have abnormal sweating, foul smelling odor or any other sweat related problem which only recently started up or which has become worse over time, you should really consult with your doctor to see if there is an underlying medical cause.

What is Sweat?

Sweating is our body's way of cooling us down. It is a clear, odorless liquid substance that can cause many people great discomfort for some people.

Sweat, or perspiration, is also one method that your body gets rid of waste matter. However, since it only does this in small amounts, the sweat glands are really used as an air conditioning system for the body.

There are about three million sweat glands all over our body. When your brain gets the signal that you're too hot, it sends a signal back telling your sweat glands to cool us down and immediately you start to perspire.

Depending on where you are, the outside conditions around you, how you're feeling and what you're doing, you will either perspire very light on certain parts of your body, or you will begin to perspire heavily.

If you have hyperhidrosis, you will perspire heavily and sometimes for no apparent reason. If you want more information about it I have gone into this in the section entitled "**Excessive Sweating (Hyperhidrosis)**".

Sometimes hyperhidrosis can be a genetic trait, but sometimes it could also be because of an underlying medical condition which prompts their body to sweat unconditionally. See a doctor if you are concerned.

The same reason can be the same as with normal sweating. If you have a foul, or offensive stench associated with your sweat, there is a possibility it is because of what you ate (i.e. curry or some strong herbs/spices). It could also be a medical issue that you will need to deal with, and the first step in doing this is to go see your doctor.

Deodorants and antiperspirants are readily available in the market to help you deal with your embarrassment to your sweating. It is the fastest remedy and simplest.

But since you're reading this book, it means that you want to a find a way out of your perspiration dilemma without having to resort to the use of such things as commercial deodorants and antiperspirants.

Don't worry, you still have a number of options open to you, but you might have to work harder at it and just walking into a convenient store and pick up a roll-on.

I can tell you here right now that the effort will be well worth it. And the very act of breaking away from mass marketed deodorants and antiperspirants is something of a relief in and of itself. It is also healthier for you!

I'm a person who prefers organic foods over non-organic foods, and who prefers to go that extra mile to get the good stuff. I wasn't always like this, there were many years in my life where I didn't really care what I put into my body, what I put on my body, and what the effects of all of these were.

Now I know better, and this is reflected in my choice of perspiration fighting agents as well. But don't get me wrong, I'm not an organic junky who thrives only on organic foods and who cringes at the thought of using any of the mass produced items that makes our lives so much easier. That is hardly the case.

I might be pickier with what I eat, but I definitely still love hamburgers and hotdogs without thinking twice sometimes. But my deodorants stay all natural.

To be honest, I've been tempted to give up my quest to find natural deodorant products. It was especially difficult when I had to go out in public without my usual deodorant and being paranoid that I'm sweating in the armpits and if I smell funny. So I won't tell you that it's going to be easy.

As I mentioned before, sweat is essentially odorless, so that although you sweat, it won't smell unless bacteria is involved.

So if you follow a simple hygiene routine of cleansing, you won't have to worry about this problem. Simple hygiene to keep odor at bay:

- Shower at least twice a day.

- Use a deodorizing or antibacterial soap.

- Wear newly washed underwear and clothes.

- Regularly wash your clothes and underwear.

- Keep excess hair trimmed or shaved under your arms where sweating excessively is a problem.

- Whenever possible either use a blow dryer to thoroughly dry out problem areas, or if you have the time allow yourself to dry out under a fan (this works!).

- Use a natural deodorant, or your own personal fragrance, or deodorizer

- Stay relaxed as much as possible. Stress can trigger an attack of intense sweating.

For more information on keeping good hygiene, de-stressing yourself, and natural deodorants, go to the section on "**Dealing with sweat naturally**".

Why do we sweat?

The maid reason we sweat is because our body needs to cool down and to get rid of toxins, but there are other reasons why we sweat.

There are so many reasons why we perspire, and some are not very common. If I take the time to list all the reasons, it would take me longer than this book to go into. There are however, a few factors which I can list that are pretty much common across the board. And these are the ones which you will find below.

- Hot weather
- Humidity
- If it's hereditary
- If you suffer from hyperhidrosis
- If you have hyperthyroidism
- Exercise or manual labor of any kind
- Stress
- Anxiety
- Embarrassment
- Medical condition/ illnesses

- It could be a reaction to certain medications you're taking

- Low blood sugar levels

- Hot/ Spicy foods

- Caffeine rich beverages

- Alcohol

- Smoking

- The onset of puberty

- Menopause

- Obesity

- Nervous dispositions

- Fever

As I said, there are many other reasons why a person sweats. Some reasons apply differently to different people. I'm sure there are reasons that we've never heard of before, but the list above is the most common ones.

We can sometimes control our sweating by controlling our emotions. The only real factors which make it difficult to control perspiration are the outside ones which are beyond our control such as adverse weather conditions, medical conditions, and genetics.

Some aspects are hard or sometimes impossible to control. For those that can be controlled, you must exert control over your bodily responses to certain situations. You need to be very string willed indeed, and have the determination to keep to your guns even if the whole world is falling down around your ears.

Don't Sweat It!

"Don't sweat it" is used often to tell someone to take it easy. The more we worry about such normal bodily functions as sweating, the more stressed we will be and the more we will sweat. Can you see where this will lead?

To be honest, I was one of those people who used to be constantly worried about my sweating when in public and also how badly I smelled. I was afraid what will people think or feel when they touch my sweaty hands or see the sweat stains on my shirt.

I stopped wearing shirts with sleeves and only black color, because although black attracts heat, it definitely didn't show the sweat marks (especially that super embarrassing round wet armpit stains!).

I started wearing lots of printed clothes and no plain colors as they show sweat more clearly. When I became tired of all the unrelieved black I did venture out in colors but mostly in dark colors or white.

When I have clammy hands, I always make sure that I either carry a handkerchief with me or that I surreptitiously wipe my hands before meeting someone. But even though I've wiped them off, my hands were still damp and cold.

I also had to use a handkerchief or something to put my hand on to avoid wetting my paper while writing.

I avoided applying any cream or lotion on my body as they tend to make my hands break out in a sweat. I washed my hands often to keep them dry.

I carried a small travel sized deodorant stick in my bag at all times. I also armed myself with wet tissue in order to wipe my armpits when they sweat. This helped me a lot.

I also enjoyed drying my underarms in the car while letting the air conditioner blow into them. The air conditioner can dry my wet pits, but it won't dry a wet shirt as fast. That is why I only wear sleeves as it is easier to only dry my armpits and not have to worry about those round wet stains on the sleeves.

These are real experiences I go through and I am not trying to lure you to read further into the book, or to appeal to your own woes.

I experienced each and every one of these just about every single day for most of my life.

It's only very recently that I have been able to overcome my deficiencies in that area, and learned to deal with things too. I am sharing my techniques deeper in the chapters below.

You might think some of my stories might not be true, but I can assure you that everything I've mention really did happen, incredible though it might sound. This also goes to illustrate how far I have come down the path to self-acceptance, and this I can say is entirely due to my experiences trying to find a way to combat my sweat problems.

That One Hot Sweaty Day

Most people are too polite to say anything or even give any indication that they have noticed your discomfort or how uncomfortable when they felt your sweaty hands, but just the thought that you are making people uncomfortable will you more to "sweat it".

At first this can be very distressing, but after a certain time you do get used to it. Since I had hyperhidrosis, summer time has always been the worst. I sweat from everywhere! My thighs, head, behind my knees were sweating buckets. I left wet foot prints around the house, and so I chose to wear house slippers to avoid myself from slipping.

There was this one time that I remember quite clearly standing out as one of the shining moments of my life. Luckily I have a sense of humor otherwise I would have been very embarrassed indeed.

The sun was blazing down on the earth and the mercury was hovering somewhere just south of 100F and it was the height of summer. Added to all of that it was a hazy day and as luck would have it, one of the few days when I had time to do my chores. This meant getting the gardening supplies, offloading the excess tools I had borrowed from a friend, and doing the shopping for the week.

The logical thing to do was for me to first drop off the tools since it was on my way, pick up the gardening supplies while the heat was still manageable and then escape with the rest of the population into the air conditioned coldness of the supermarket when the heat was at its worst.

I went along doing my tasks and it was only when I arrived at the supermarket that I found everybody had had the same idea as me, and we were squeezed in tighter than in a tin of sardines!

I was tempted to put off shopping for another day, but I really wasn't looking forward to another night of microwavable food especially not when I was in the grocery and had the ability to pick up my own pizza fixings.

And this, ladies and gentlemen, is where things took an unexpected twist. Like I said it was a lucky thing I have thick skin and can find the humor in most situations.

It was while I was in the snacks aisle choosing what chips I would buy that I encountered a woman staring at me behind her cart with a strange disapproving stare on her face. I couldn't figure it out if I actually knew her or even what I had done wrong to warrant that disapproving stare, so I just went on choosing my chips.

To cut a long story short, her two kids came around the aisle towards me, and the surprise came when the woman uttered a sharp command to the children to get away from me! I was surprised to say the least and could only stare back - after all, what had I done?

I only realized the reason when she sniffed and marched out of the supermarket with her two kids in tow, that she was offended by the sight of the sweat stains on my shirt, as well as by the sweat that was only just cooling on it me.

I giggled a little and shook my head. I was amused by the whole episode and when I turned back to my chips to find other people staring at what had just happened, I could only smile harder in response. It was the first time I had come up against a strong prejudice against the body's natural cooling function.

What's even funnier was that most of the shoppers there were in a similar condition to me since the air conditioning in the supermarket had apparently given up the fight to stay alive and just took a summer vacation.

What's worse, even the store employees working heavy crates of fruits and vegetables back and forth were covered in perspiration. It was an unavoidable condition given the type of day it was and the dead air conditioner. The whole situation is nothing we should sweat about.

But I thought of sharing this story with you, not to highlight the absurd behavior of the woman in the supermarket, but the fact that it really does take all sorts to make the world turn around, and no matter where you go, or what you do you will always encounter someone of her ilk.

To that end, it is best if you develop a thick skin to such unwarranted barbs and go about your business as usual.

But what you really need to take away from this little encounter out of my past, is that the only way you can be comfortable with your sweaty issues, is if you are comfortable within yourself.

Let's accept the fact that sweating is natural and that sometimes (like when it's a hundred degrees outside, hazy and hot), it's necessary to sweat. In fact you should be slightly worried if you don't sweat in those types of conditions. There must be something wrong and I recommend you go see your physician.

Sometimes it could be embarrassing or inappropriate socially to go out in public drenched in sweat, but experience in the supermarket I was talking about was definitely not one of those times. I have accepted that there will be people who will not accept it, and that's alright. There is after all, only so much of staying-fresh that you can do in the middle of a heat wave!

What to do about it?

After all said and done, now, I'm going to give you a few quick tips to dealing with sweat and odor *after* you've drenched yourself with perspiration. Why? Because this section is almost as important as learning how to stay sweat and odor free.

I'm not giving any fast and immediate cure methods here on how to stop sweating. Everything that I have mentioned in this book will take time to work. Also keep in mind that your body metabolism is different to mine, and for another thing it will take some time for your body to throw off the yoke of dependence upon the deodorants and antiperspirants that you've been using to date. Give it some time.

A good example is the length of time it took me to be able to properly use a natural deodorant, like the ones I've mentioned later on.

It always seemed like it was working because for the first few days the natural deodorant would do as good a job as my antiperspirant, but pretty much after about the first week to week and a half it would stop working.

After many a trial and errors of trying various different natural remedies, I came to the realization that I would need to stop using my normal antiperspirant/deodorant stick completely if I hoped to have any chance for the natural treatments to work. Eek!

I don't promise miracles in this book; what you will get instead, are down to earth and practical ideas which you can use to get away from chemical based commercial deodorants/antiperspirants can control your sweating naturally.

The Quick Fix

These are a few things that you can do to make your life easier while making the transition from normal deodorants and antiperspirants to natural deodorants and antiperspirants.

So here are a few "quick fixes" you've been looking for.

Bear in mind that these are only quick fixes. They won't fix any sweat or odor complaints that you have on any kind of long term basis, but they are heaven-sent when you need a quick pick me up. They are simple and you can start right now!

Carry a handkerchief around with you

If you sweat at all different times of the day and at the most inconvenient times as well, you should always carry a small handkerchief around with you. Carry more than one if you know you will be doing many activities going outdoors.

A pack of wet tissues will be very handy too. They are not just cooling and refreshing, but they can also take away bacteria that cause odor.

Drink plenty of water

This should be a no-brainer really, but some people seem to think that if they drink less water that they will sweat less. If it were that easy we would all have given up on water and water based drinks long ago to control our sweating.

We need water to live, and if we tend to perspire heavily and don't replenish our water reserves, we will most likely fall prey to dehydration. Keep yourself hydrated when you sweat a lot. Bring a water bottle if you need to do so.

The standard amount of water you need is about 6-8 glasses is the recommended minimum amount of water we need to drink, and watch as your health takes a swing for the better. Your skin will clear up and even your hair will be healthier.

Avoid spicy foods

This doesn't necessarily apply to everyone out there. Some of us are quite used to eating spicy on a daily basis and indeed, some people need it as part of their daily dietary requirements.
Unfortunately for someone like myself and probably others, just a little spicy food can jumpstart my metabolic rate and making me hotter, and ultimately leading me to sweat.

Do you feel sweat beading on your forehead and above your lips when you decide to treat yourself to that wonderful takeout of hot and spicy Thai salad?

Or maybe that zesty chicken curry you tried the other day when you went for lunch with your friends? Remember also the gallons of iced water you drank just to keep your sweating impulses under wraps?

Some foods and ingredients just have that effect on some people, and the best way to deal with this is to know your own boundaries and limitations. I also tend to have an upset stomach when I eat food that is very spicy.

If you tend break into a sweat when you eat hot or spicy foods, then avoid them when you're in social situations where you want to stay dry. Instead, reserve those foods as a treat for when you're at home with the family or when you're alone.

Stay out of the heat

This might be the easiest advice to avoid sweating, but it's definitely one of those things that many of us ignore.

Yes, we know that it's hot. Yes, we know that we're prone to heat stroke, sunburn and excessive sweating when exposed to hot temperatures. But do we exercise our right to survive and get out of the heat? No.

Why? Not realizing exactly how hot it is, or we think that we're strong enough to withstand a small heat wave can be dangerous. Most times we just don't realize how dangerously hot it is until we're drenched in sweat and perhaps light headed.

Always pay attention to your sweat glands. If it's hotter than you can handle you can be certain that your sweat glands will go into overdrive to help you cool off. That's what they are there for: to help our body regulate its temperature.

It doesn't mean you should be indoor all the time, just try and get into some shade. Do anything to help you cool off and your sweat glands to come back to normal such as have a drink of water or a cool wet towel can immediately relieve your body from the heat.

Mind over sweat

This one might take some time to master, but is something that most of us can utilize without anyone being the wiser for it.

Using imagery of a cool place, or imagining yourself in the middle of a warm breeze can help you to bring down your inner temperature, which will in turn bring your sweat response back into a proper balance.

This will take a little practice to get this right, but it does work. My favorite image is riding alongside the beach with the car's top down and the salty wind washing over me.

The other thing that you can try is meditation to help regulate your body temperature, but this one will definitely take a lot of practice.

Take a swim (not a hike!)

If you have access to a pool or any kind of water that's good for a dip, this is one of the better ideas. If you're stuck in office or at home with no way to get yourself down to a large cooling body of water to take a much needed swim, then this particular quick fix can be frustrating.

Other than that tiny glitch in your world, if you can find a way to cool off using water for purposes other than drinking, I say take it! If you can swim, then take a swim. If you can have a cooling shower, then go for it. Don't forget to apply sunblock!

Wear light and loose clothing

This is also a no-brainer, but do you how many times that I personally have gone outside wearing thick heavy tight-fitting clothing? It's too many times to even count. And I know for a fact that I'm not the only person to have done this either.

Skin tight clothing which lies like a second skin against your skin is definitely not the way to go about staying sweat free. It might look good initially, but how good do you look with large sweat stains on your clothes?

So wear loose fitting clothing so that you won't overly sweat, and so that you get proper ventilation on your body.

Another course of action you can take is to wear a plain white cotton t-shirt beneath your shirts or blouses. Some people find this to be very helpful in stopping the action of sweat reaching your outer clothes, but I'm one of those people who finds that it causes me to sweat even more vigorously!

Don't attract heat

What do I mean by that? Dark colored clothing attracts heat. So wear light colors to go along with the loose fitting clothing I mentioned in the earlier section. This might be elementary knowledge for many people, but truly how many of us follow what we know is right?

Wear whites, or reds, or blues, or greens, but stay away from the black!

Use those baby wipes

Work it baby! Use those baby wipes like there's no tomorrow.
Actually, use only one or two and that only when the need arises. And when I say 'need' I'm talking about when you're sweating so much that your new loose flowing silk blouse looks as if it was molded on to your skin!

Having a small packet of baby wipes or even a small packet of wet tissues with you comes in handy. You can always take a quick to the restroom where you can wedge yourself firmly into a stall and wipe away the perspiration using the towelettes.

The towelettes also have the added benefit of cleansing the sweat affected areas so that it's almost as if you took a shower! And depending on whether you bought the scented variety or the unscented variety, you will also have a nice fresh scent clinging to you.

For added freshness and protection, if you also take along your natural deodorant or other convenient travel sized sweat- and odor-fighting item, you can apply it after you wipe your sweat off with the wipes.

At this point you might be thinking that you don't really want to have to carry all of these things with you everywhere you go.

But the fact of the matter is, that until you can find a viable natural method to deal with your perspiration problems, using these little tips, even this one, is the best way to live your life free of any embarrassing sweaty moments.

Stay away from caffeine

If caffeine is needed in the morning to get you moving and functioning, then by all means go ahead with it, but I would suggest you cut it down to just the one cup in the morning, and not an entire pot!

"Why??" you might ask. Coffee has the added bonus of stimulating your body and raising your metabolic rate. And after all, this is the reason you need your shot of caffeine in the morning isn't it, to help you rejoin the human race?

Having more than one cup of caffeine when you know that you get revved up is just committing a cardinal no-sweat sin. Drinking a pot of coffee, or other caffeine laden beverage into your system, you're telling your body that it's all right to sweat because you need to boost your metabolism. So keep it to a minimal.

Go bare!

No, I don't mean for you to go in your birthday suit. If Mother Nature intended us to go around in our altogether she most definitely would not have provided us with cotton bushes, silk worms, lambs, and a naturally inquisitive and inventive mind.

So, no, I'm not asking you to join a nudist's colony. I'm talking about those all important pair of stockings, pantyhose or leggings which most women feel is a must, when stepping out of the house.

And if it's not any of these, you can bet your bottom dollar that it will be in the form of jeans, shorts, or even loose fitting trousers. Although the latter isn't so bad, you can do so much better than this!

Times were when a woman wouldn't think twice about wearing a dress or a skirt. Now, it's the exception more than the norm. This has, in its own way brought about its problems.

And the one that concerns us now is the fact that none of this attire aids in keeping you sweat free. Every single last one of them, with perhaps the exception of the loose flowing trousers, only adds to your discomfort and encourages your body to sweat more.

Yes, even the shorts can make you feel hot, especially tight fitting shorts that leave no room for your skin to breathe. The best thing that you could do for yourself right now, would be to lose the 'hose, the stockings, the leggings, the jeans and whatever other type of cover up you have for your legs.

Instead go bare. Wear skirts instead of jeans and ditch the 'hose. There's nothing more attractive than a woman wearing a skirt, and there is no 'hose lines showing, what you get is sheer beauty. That's for the onlooker.

What you personally get out of losing your normal leg-covering attire is the peace of mind that comes with knowing you won't be sweating gallons.

You feel comfortable, you know you look good, and there's nothing to beat the feel of a cool breeze on bare legs that have been forever cooped up in some type of covering or other.

Put your right foot forward

One of the best ways to keep your feet odor and sweat free is to put your best foot forward. Wear well ventilated shoes and watch as the odor causing germs just vanish.

Keeping your feet covered, in a more than likely cramped pair of shoes, and you will find yourself suffering for it. It will feel highly uncomfortable when your feet are wet and not able to get dry inside those stuffy shoes.

Or if you find that you can't always wear a comfortable pair of sandals or open toed shoes, and that you need to always keep your feet enclosed in a pair of sweat-inducing dress shoes or trainers, then take whatever time you have to yourself, to slip your feet out of those shoes.

Of course if you have an odor issue with your feet then the last thing that you want to do will be to take your shoes off in the middle of a public area, but if you do have somewhere you can go for some privacy and five or ten minutes to spare, then I would strongly suggest that you give your feet a break from the burden of having to wear shoes.

Find a small bottle of normal talcum powder or foot powder with you to put on your beleaguered feet. You can also buy one of travel size foot sprays. This can give your feet much needed relief, and will also keep the odor and sweating down to a minimum.

Alternately you could take along a second pair of shoes with you. This can also help to minimize sweating problems, and also gives your feet time to air out in a nice clean pair of shoes.

Re-hydrate if you're dehydrated

This is common sense, but sometimes in the middle of things we fail to notice it until it's too late.

If you're going to be outdoor for some time, then the best thing that you can do for yourself would be to carry a bottle of water or a sports drink around with you.

Sometimes I drink a sports drink when I sweat a whole lot. This will replenish the water, and the salts and minerals you're losing through your sweat.
But it doesn't even have to be a hot day, and you don't even have to be in the hot sun to become dehydrated.

If you have left it till the last minute and you can feel yourself fading away or light headed, quickly guzzle down some glucose enriched water, or a sports drink. This will replenish your depleted stores of minerals and salt. An electrolyte can also be useful.

If you're like me and are prone to sweating in any condition, then you can become dehydrated. You need to stay on top of this and always keep replenishing your body with liquids.

If you can't find any sports drink or electrolyte, but you do have access to your kitchen, (or anyone else's kitchen for that matter), you can use this quick fix to get yourself back on your feet.

- Dilute 1 teaspoon of Apple Cider Vinegar into a glass of cool water (not iced), and drink it down. This will replenish the depleted stores of salt and minerals in your body.

A cup of tea?

"What? A hot cup of tea in this heat?" you might ask. Yes, and not iced tea either. You might think this is insane, but this is one little secret that I know works.

You might need some time to get used to this idea, but when you get into the habit it quickly becomes the highlight of your day. The tea, when drunk while still hot, is refreshing, and even though you might find that you sweat a little initially, it helps to cool you down.

So the next time you're looking for some liquid to refresh yourself from the heat, stay away from the coffee and the sodas, and take the time off to sit down and take a relaxing cup of tea. The benefits are twofold as you will find that the time you spend over your cup of tea also relaxing.

Excessive Sweating (Hyperhidrosis)

More people than you know might be suffering from hyperhidrosis. I am one of them. In fact more people than even they themselves are aware, might be suffering from hyperhidrosis.

Hyperhidrosis is a state where you tend to sweat more than normal, most common of the palms, armpits and soles. For many people this is a very distressing problem. Although some people who have hyperhidrosis sweat only marginally more than normal, most sufferers of hyperhidrosis perspire heavily.

And this need not only be when they are in conditions which will make them perspire, for example doing hard labor, exercising, going out in the hot sun etc.

People who suffer from hyperhidrosis will tend to sweat excessively in most cases, no matter where they are or what they are doing. For me, just eating dinner or watching a movie can trigger sweating.

For others, just moving a stack of magazines from the coffee table to the floor can bring on an attack of sweating. It's different from person to person.

These are the very extreme cases of hyperhidrosis, but they are also becoming more and more common. The first thing that you need to do if you believe yourself to be suffering from hyperhidrosis is to consult your doctor or other medical professional.

There could be an underlying medical cause for your excessive sweating, other than genes. If this is the case then the sooner you learn what your body is trying to tell you, the better. It can also help your peace of mind to rule out any medical cause. Sometimes the stress of worrying can bring on bouts of intense sweating.

Also if you only just recently started to have signs of hyperhidrosis, it's always helpful to find out whether your body is going through a perfectly normal change or whether you need to change something in your lifestyle to get back on track.

Some people prefer to treat their hyperhidrosis with drugs or even the more radical and permanent method of surgery, but there can be alternatives to either of these approaches.

In most cases of hyperhidrosis, normally antiperspirants don't work, and it sure didn't work for me. Your only option may seem like taking sweat inhibiting medications, injections, or using the surgical methods (like I did).

But if you are willing to suffer for your cause a little bit longer and you don't expect miracles, you might be able to find a remedy for your sweating problems through natural means.

Even people who do not suffer from hyperhidrosis wish to get away from the chemical enriched world of store bought deodorants and antiperspirants are now looking for more natural methods with which to control their sweating. You are one of them as you are reading this book.

These methods, many of which I have mentioned in this book, can work, but the same method that worked for your friend won't necessarily work for you. You will have to go through a few methods before finding the right method for you.

And although some of these methods might seem too "soft" and not work for hyperhidrosis sufferers, they all have the ability to work for you, but first of all, you need to acknowledge that you do have hyperhidrosis, and you also need to eliminate that you might be caused by a medical condition.

When you have gone through these steps you can then go about finding a natural sweat prevention method to deal with your hyperhidrosis.

It will take time however, and sometimes you will find that you have to go through more than one treatment method to find the one that suits you, but it can be done. You can be rid of excessive perspiration and do it in a natural manner as well.

Where we sweat

Not everyone is aware of this, but many of us in fact, sweat not only under our arms but also on our scalp, genital area, hands, feet, back, neck and forehead.

These are of course the most common places on the body where people can sweat, and of these the most common are the underarms and the genital/ groin area.

No one is built exactly alike and this means that no one sweats alike either. A person, who perspires on their hands and feet, won't necessarily have the same sweating dripping off their hands and feet like I used to have.

Yes, dripping like as if I just took a shower.

There are also times when a person suffering from hyperhidrosis might not perspire from their armpits.

It is possible for a person to sweat excessively from their facial area, or their torso and armpits, and sweat only normally elsewhere. This in itself is very disturbing and can cause much emotional distress. Not to mention embarrassing.

If you think about it, it can't be very easy to be socially active when your palms are always sweaty and damp, or when you have sweat dripping down the sides of your face when you're in an air conditioned room.

It is very difficult to deal with excessively sweaty feet when you have to be constantly wearing shoes. Just the not so appealing odor alone is enough to cause anyone distress, and when it's paired with the other problems you can get as a result of constantly damp feet, it puts things into a whole new perspective.

This is why hyperhidrosis in any form is distressing to anyone who suffers from it.

And unless genetics plays a big part in your hyperhidrosis problems then the first thing that you will want to do is to go ahead and make an appointment with your doctor or physician.

You can then eliminate whether or not you have any medical problems which might lead to your having hyperhidrosis. Another thing that you might want to take into account is whether your excessive sweating problems began only recently or whether they were longstanding.

All of these counts when you're deciding what type of action to take against your problem and a clear understanding of all of these will help you immeasurably.

The different forms of hyperhidrosis:

- **Primary Hyperhidrosis** -- this is when a person sweats excessively without a known cause

- **Secondary Hyperhidrosis** -- there is a cause for the excessive sweating, and it is mostly medical in nature

- **Axillary Hyperhidrosis** -- this type of excessive sweating is the most normally occurring type

- **Facial Hyperhidrosis** -- this is where a person has excessive sweating on the facial area, scalp area, and they may even have severe blushing

- **Palmer Hyperhidrosis** -- this is when you experience excessive sweating on the palm of your hands

- **Plantar Hyperhidrosis** -- sweating occurs on the soles of your feet, and also in between your toes, and can in turn lead to fungal infections if the area is not cleaned properly and aired on a daily basis

- **Truncal Hyperhidrosis** -- sweat occurs on the thigh area, and the genital/ groin area

Should you see the doctor?

As I mentioned earlier, when you have hyperhidrosis, or if you think you suffer from hyperhidrosis, you really should see the doctor about it. But how do you know whether you need to go see your doctor or not?

Some people are not comfortable talking about such a potentially embarrassing subject as excessive sweating.

This is really when you need to be aware of your body and be aware of how your body works.

Everyone might have the same general and overall bodily functions, but each individual will function in a different way, and just because your father, mother, brother or sister function in one way, that doesn't mean that your body will function in the same manner.

This is why if you know your body and are self aware of how your body normally works, you can tell immediately if there is a difference such as excessive sweating.

So when should you go see your doctor?

- If you only recently started to sweat excessively where before you were sweating normally.

- If you notice a foul or offensive smell emanating from your sweat.

  Sweat in and of itself is odorless; it's only when it interacts with the bacteria on your skin that you notice an odor.

- If your sweating becomes a problem for you socially and inhibits your free interaction in society as a whole

- If your sweating embarrasses you and causes you considerable discomfort

- If you experience recurrent fever or dizziness, or even a rapid heartbeat in association with your sweating

- If you sweat even when you're in a situation which normally wouldn't make a person sweat, like being in an air conditioned room

- If your sweat irritates your skin

- If it has an abnormal color

A few things we can do

In this section I thought I would give you a short list of the things that you can do to help you either prevent sweating, or deal with odor problems. Each and every one of the items I have mentioned here, I have also mentioned in greater detail in the section "Dealing with Sweat Naturally".

I've only mentioned them here so that you can get a head start on the things that you need to do in order to stay sweat and odor free.

These are only a few practical tips and suggestions to get you started on your journey to finding a natural sweat prevention measure.

Drink plenty of water

You might think that this might give you the opposite result that you might want to achieve; after all if you sweat a lot you don't want to give your body more ammunition to embarrass you some more, right? Wrong.

If you sweat a lot (and even if you don't), then water is your number one best friend. Without it you could become severely dehydrated without your even being aware of it. See the section on "Water" for more information.

Wear the right clothing

This might be common sense to some people, but quite a lot of us still wear all the wrong types of clothing and can't figure out what's going wrong.

The trick with your clothes is to avoid such sweat inducing fabrics such as clothes made from non-natural fibers such as nylon. You need to wear natural fiber clothing such as cotton clothes.

Cotton is the best alternative you have to help you stay cool. Avoid silks and heavy-weights like wool. They are natural but they can also make you sweat - to put it indelicately - like a pig!

In fact, although that new silk blouse you bought might look great on you now, before your day is even done you will find that you are either soaking or have great big sweat stain rings under your arms.

Another thing that you'll want to look out for in your clothing is whether or not you're wearing tight fitting clothing or loose clothing. For instance, tight fitting clothing will make it difficult for the sweat to dry out whereas wearing loose fitting clothing will help the air to circulate and your sweat to dry off faster.

Then again you will need to look into the color of your clothing as well, and to find out about this and more about the various clothing you should wear go to the section entitled "Clothing".

Proper Hygiene

I cannot say too much on this subject, and although many people take care of the most basic of hygiene essentials, some of the elements of hygiene are not necessarily given the number one priority spot.

To that end, although I probably don't need to say it, I will. There are a few things which you need to do to have good hygiene and this encompasses so much more than merely showering on a daily basis.

I have covered this in more detail in the section marked "Good Hygiene" but here are a few of the more basic ones that you might want to look into.

- Daily/ regular bathing or showering
- Regular change of clothes

- Regularly washing clothes -- it's no use changing clothes once or twice a day if you go and wear the same sweat soaked-and-dried t-shirt again tomorrow!

- Usage of soap or other like products

Change your Diet

I will not go into many details on this subject, so I will keep things short and sweet here so that you don't become bored when you get to the meat and bones of the section later on under the section headed "Proper Diet".

What I do want to clarify before going any further is that when I talk about changing your diet, I'm not only talking about changing your diet to a more healthier option.

Literally I'm talking about your diet here and now because sometimes the foods you eat could be a factor in your sweating problems as well any odor problems that you might have.

For instance eating or overeating things like:

- Garlic
- Onions
- Fish
- Curry
- or even Red meats

These things can give your perspiration a bad odor. If this is one of your major battles, then one of the first things you will want to do is to rule out food as your major odor or sweat causer.

After that if things don't look up, in fact if they keep going steadily downhill from there, you should look into getting a medical diagnosis to definitely rule out any underlying medical conditions which may be causing your sweating or bad odor.

Alcohol

This is one thing that many people will find hard to give up, but it can help in the battle against sweat and odor. Giving up not only alcohol but cigarettes as well, can help especially if are in the habit of taking both far in excess of what is good for you.

In fact you don't need to give up alcohol or smoking entirely, but if you can find it within you to cut down on excessive amounts of either, you will go a long way towards helping yourself.

And it's not only that, things like caffeine rich beverages and products can also have an adverse reaction on you and may cause you to sweat. To learn more on this subject you might want to check out the section I've marked separately for this called, "Alcohol, Coffee, and Smoking".

Hot Flashes

This is not something new and most women will experience at least one in their lifetime. I say "most women" here because not all women will experience hot flashes, or even experience it to such a degree that they feel discomfort.

Hot flashes can be very uncomfortable and in some cases even close to debilitating for some women. Hot flashes are also one reason for excessive or even abnormal sweating.

What I mean by abnormal sweating is sweating that is out of sync with your normal sweating habits. First of all, you must realize and recognize that you are having hot flashes.

Some women get such severe hot flashes that they might even feel as if they are having a heart attack.

This of course, is the more serious and debilitating type of hot flash. How severe and regularity which women experience differ from one person to the next.

I won't cover the reasons for a person getting hot flashes, here. That's a book all by itself and since this book is about sweating I thought we might continue with that trend of thought instead!

The reason I bought up the subject of hot flashes though was because sweating can be caused when a person experiences a hot flash, and this most definitely falls into my realm of what to do and what not to do.

Therefore below, I've outlined a few things that you can do to curb sweating or how to deal with the sudden drenching that you might get. But the best thing that I can say is to follow the simple guidelines I've given in the book to staying cool and dealing with excessive sweating.

What you can do about it

What you will find in this section will be detailed more deeply in the section on "**Dealing with sweat naturally**", but sometimes it helps to have the information where you can find it most easily.

If you were having a hot flash, or could feel one pending then the very last thing that you would want to do would be to have to flip through or read the entire section on what to do, when you want answers, Now!

So, here it is, to give you a quick help. If you want more answers you can go to the section on how to deal naturally with your sweat which I mentioned earlier, or you can even go to the section called **"What you can to do about it".**

This section is another quick-fix for those of you who are impatient and don't want to read through the entire natural remedies section when you are sweating purposely.

The things I've mentioned below won't help you to shake loose your hot flash symptoms for ever and ever; they're designed mainly to help you get through your trying times.

As I said hot flashes are a separate book by itself, and I'm afraid the treatment for it also falls into the same category.

Take a cold shower

No, this is not a joke. If you have the time and the ability to do so, you should take a cold shower if you're in a place to do so. Or better still, if you have the time indulge yourself with a nice long soak in lukewarm water.

The trick here is not to lay in either extreme of water since laying in hot water will make your hot flash worse, and lying in cold water will only make you shiver!

De-stress and relax

Being overly stressed or anxious is one of the reasons you might be experiencing hot flashes, so take a little "me" time, even ten minutes away from the home or office taking a calming walk around the block can help.

If you feel a hot flash coming on, and you know that part of the problem is you're stressed condition, trying to find those ten minutes can be a heaven-sent way of dealing with the hot flash.

If however, you find that hot flash coming on just before a meeting, or while you're in a meeting, you will need to resort to a few mind tricks.

The easiest is using meditation to help you deal with it, but if you don't know how or you're just beginning to learn, you can try the alternative to deep meditation, which is using imagery.

Imagine yourself in a cool place, maybe a beach, maybe the freezer, whichever works. All you need is a "cool place" for you to go to.

Of course sometimes this might not work for you, in which case, you will need to resort to the old standby of drinking water. I don't recommend something too cold or filled with ice; you will almost definitely feel hotter after gulping down ice cold water. Just a normal room temperature drink or two will do wonders for you.

Always keep water handy

If you're prone to hot flashes and intensive bouts of sweating, then keeping a small bottle of water handy with you is one of the best ways you can do for dealing with your unexpected sweating.

If water is not the thing for you, then keep something like a sports drink with you. Any type of beverage such as fruit juice is also good; anything isn't caffeine laden. You would want to stay away from is coffee, it can increase your sweating, not help you with it.

Stay in wide open places

If you can. This is not always possible especially if you're on the 34th floor of your office building with no way to get to that cooling, green park you know is only a few blocks away.

If you could, get out from your office or from anywhere you're cooped up inside. If you have the time, go for a relaxing drive away from the bustling business of the city.

Whatever you do, do not go for a drive in the city; you will probably get more aggro and start sweating more intensely. Your stress levels will also peak!

Avoid synthetic fiber clothing

I've mentioned it before and I will keep mentioning it throughout the book. If you know you sweat a lot, or if you don't want to sweat a lot, then avoid wearing clothing made from synthetic fibers!

- Wear natural fiber clothing such as cottons, linens, and in winter time silks and wools.

- Dress in layers. Whether you're wearing wools and silks for winter, or cottons and linens for summer, dress in layers. You know that you get hot flashes, and you know you can never predict when exactly you will get a hot flash, at least not until a few minutes beforehand, so dress in layers.

This way you can remove one garment at a time according to the degree of discomfort you're feeling. Obviously there's only so far that you can go, and only in some places where you can do this, but it always helps to be prepared.

Use a fan

Keep a small battery operated fan with you to use whenever possible if you have no recourse to an air-conditioner or thermostat unit.

Even a paper fan will do, and these can be found quite cheaply at knick knack stores, or you can even make your own paper fan, like you did when you were a kid.

Just in case you didn't here's how: Take a sheet of blank paper, keep it lengthwise in front of you, and starting from one short side fold in an accordion manner until the entire paper is folded.

Voila, you now have you own quick and easy fan, and all you have to do is grasp the two outer edges and unfurl slightly to reveal your fan.

Let's Stop the Sweating

This is the part that you've really been waiting for. All those little snippets of information have only whetted your appetite and fueled your determination to find a natural remedy to deal with your perspiration problems.

If you're tired of hearing about these, and you want to go on to the section of **"Dealing with sweat naturally"**, feel free to skip ahead. This is only a brief overview of what all your options are.

Through conventional means

As I said in the earlier section, this is only to give you an overview of your options for dealing with sweat and sweat-produced odor. So if you decide that you want to go with these options after all and leave the natural methods for the birds, you will need to dig around for more information using other means.

And one of the better places to find information on these will be from your doctor. He/ she will normally be able to tell you which methods are suitable for you.

But for most people who prefer to stay with the more conventional methods, the antiperspirants and deodorants which line the grocery store, and drug store shelves, are your easiest options.

The other options listed here are either drastic measures, and/ or very costly. So you will need to weigh your options carefully.

Antiperspirants and Deodorants

The one thing that you probably didn't know about these was that the FDA classes antiperspirants as drugs. That's right, they class them as drugs, obviously not on the same scale as such things as mind controlling drugs, but under the classification of drugs (read: medications, here) which alter your body or your body chemistry in some way.

Deodorants are classed as cosmetics and don't come under the same strict rules and regulations that antiperspirants do. Even so, in my book this makes both of them equally bad.

On the one hand, you have a product whose ingredients need to be approved as safe for usage by humans, and on the other hand, you have a product that requires very little approval on what ingredients it presents in its product.

After all that have been said, these are the products which are readily available for us to use, and it behooves me to tell you what functions they serve.

Antiperspirant works prevents the sweat glands on your body from functioning. The main ingredient is Aluminum Chlorohydrate which works on us by partially blocking the pores so that sweat cannot come through.

Deodorants don't prevent you from sweating. Their function is entirely different from antiperspirants. They cause no change in your body. Instead, deodorants work to eliminate odor. This is why deodorants have been classed in the cosmetic range, because it only works on a superficial level.

Most people believe deodorants to do the same job as antiperspirants, but this is just not the case. That's why if you pick up a deodorant by accident at the supermarket you will come home to find out that it doesn't work in stopping you from sweating.

Surgical Methods

Surgical methods make permanent changes to your body and inhibiting your sweat glands completely. This is a very radical step, so you really need to think hard about it before you have this procedure done.

Talk with your doctor about all your options, and if you want, you might also think about getting some counseling. Sweat can be a very serious issue if you have suffered because of it for most of your life, and although this might seem like the best way to deal with it, you will want to think hard on it before going through with it.

Also, talking with someone who is not part of your life, like a counselor or therapist or your doctor, will generally help you to get things in perspective. Just remember that once this surgery is performed it isn't reversible.

There is also the little matter of side effects which you can get as a result of this surgery, and these you will definitely to know about beforehand. Make sure that you have all your facts before going in for surgery and make sure that you are one hundred percent sure that this is what you want.

Botox Injections

No, this is not for you to have plastic surgery or to ease out the wrinkles under your arms. It has been shown that injecting the Botulinum toxin into you can stop your sweat glands from producing sweat for weeks or even months on end.

The bad part about it? Besides the fact that you're injecting something into your body with the word "toxin" affixed to it, it costs an arm and a leg to have this procedure done on a regular basis.

Dealing with Sweat Naturally

There are many ways you can deal with sweat naturally without resorting to the usual products in the market that contain chemicals and things. For different people this can be for a number of reasons, but for me personally it began when I started to get adverse reactions to my deodorants and antiperspirants such as itchiness and burning sensations.

It took me some time to win the war of the sweats, and in that time I did vacillate between natural deodorants and my normal up-to-then used antiperspirant/deodorant.

I struggled between wanting to get rid of my allergic reactions, to wanting to stay fresh smelling throughout the day without having to worry about what other people would think (or smell) when I walked by or stood next to them.

Obviously, it was not a good time for me, and to compound matters I also started to sweat more through my scalp, but this coincided with a temporary move I had to make to warmer climes.

When I moved back home that problem got better, but I still had other issues I had to deal with and so far nothing I was doing was working properly for me. Frustration came along.

It took me a while to see the fact, but when I did it made so much sense to me. I was left wondering why I hadn't seen it before.

I was staring me in the face was I've missed all along. It has been in front of my face and in my face most of my life. To mix a metaphor, I couldn't see the tree for the forest!

So what is this unveiled fact I found? Diet.

As simple as that. Well, it wasn't "simple" by any means, but it was the writing on the wall which I had been ignoring having been inundated with it.

Diet wasn't and isn't the one secret that can get you back on track and on your way to a sweat- and odor-free lifestyle. But it sure can help.

Your diet will help bring your body back into its natural balance so that the other natural deodorizing methods you're using, have a better chance to work.

Naturally it will not be immediate and it will take a few months for your change in diet to be reflected in your sweat problems. But if you keep it up, you will be surprised at the outcome.

Again, I would like to say this again, I'm not a doctor and I don't advocate any type of medical changes or course of medications for your sweat problems.

I am just presenting a number of different methods which I have used, to deal with my own sweat problems. Please chose which ones you think will work for you and don't forget to consult with your doctor first.

I've mentioned that I do not claim that changing your diet is the best course of action for you to take. Especially in the case where you are on medication, or where you are on a specialized diet, you should first consult with your doctor before making any changes in your diet or lifestyle.

For me personally, diet was part of the treatment and not the entire treatment itself.

Before we proceed, you should also note that not everyone will react in the same way to different sweat prevention and deodorizing methods.

We are all different. Different people have different body balances and they will react differently. So although what worked for me, might not work for you. Trial and error will be needed to find the best ones for you.

Remember that just because something is natural that it doesn't mean it's good for anyone and everyone. Some people are allergic to natural things such as plants and some type of seafood. My favorite example here is shellfish.

It's all-natural, right? And many people love to eat shellfish like prawns, but there are also a number of people who are allergic to prawns and can't go anywhere near them.

This entire section is devoted to the pursuit of finding what works and if you go through it you will find a number of suggestions on what you can do.

I have mentioned a few of these things in the beginning of the book. I just want to say that even though I might go between a few remedies, there are a few core things that I do on a daily basis which I believe help me to keep on the right track.

These are, in no particular order:

- Healthy diet

- Good hygiene
- Wearing the right clothes

Everything else to me is secondary and just goes to controlling or minimizing sweat or odor. By following these four basics I have found the right combination of factors to use in staying embarrassment- and sweat stain-free.

Good Hygiene

This is very simple and I've mentioned it before. I'll try and keep it short and sweet, but most definitely to the point.

Shower daily

- Showering daily and at least twice a day is a great way to help you cope with sweat.

- If you suffer from excessive sweat then sometimes you might need to shower up to three times a day, but if you feel the need to go beyond that you might either want to consult with your doctor, or you might want to find a better sweat remedy to go along with your daily cleansing routine.

Use a deodorizing soap

- Use a deodorizing soap or better still, an antibacterial soap.

- Many people will tell you that using soap is bad for you and the overall pH balance of your skin, and I have to say that I do agree with them. Using too much soap is bad for you, but then again anything will be bad for you when overused.

- The key here is moderation. Use soap by all means, but don't use a complete bar during one or two showers. Use it sparingly, especially the harsher soaps as they will strip the skin of all of its natural oils.

- Ideally I would advocate that you get to the stage where you can either go without soap, or use it only very minimally almost as if it were the last bar of soap on earth and you would never see another one again as long as you lived.

Exfoliate

- Whether you use a loofah to do so, or whether you use a body scrub to do so, you need to exfoliate.

- Don't be too harsh on your skin when exfoliating, but give yourself a good scrub anyway. This removes the layer of dead cells from your skin, and takes with it a layer of odor causing bacteria. It also helps to take away the residue of whatever product, or natural deodorizer you've used.

This is really good whether you're using natural products or whether you're using chemical based antiperspirants.

When my underarm started to hurt in localized place I knew that I was close to getting a blister, so I would know that I had to start using my loofah immediately.

I didn't do this every time until I became used to it. I showered and really it was only until then that I needed to be get to the loofah before the blisters got to me.

- Use loofah once or twice a week. Body scrub can also be used.

Tip: I have found that face scrub is gentler on sensitive skin, and it does the same job. But just to be on the safe side is why I make regular use of the loofah.

Wear newly washed clothes

There's absolutely no use in your taking a shower if the moment you step out of it, you step into your old sweat stained clothes. This kind of defeats the purpose and will only send you back into odor-land once more, rendering moot the time you took to have a shower.

- It's simple really, take a shower, dry off, use your natural deodorant, and then step into a clean set of clothes.

- If you don't wash your clothes on a regular and frequent basis, then you'll be finding yourself in for a nasty surprise when you can't stay odor free!

- If you don't sweat like a pig, then you can always go out on a limb and wear the same clothes about two to three days, but that really should be the maximum number of days that you step into the same set of clothes.

Tip: Wear newly laundered clothes as often as possible.

Regularly wash your clothes

This should be obvious, but some people have dredged out something that was only marginally unclean from our washing baskets when we forgot to do the washing for the week? We all know that we are guilty of this.

- By not regularly washing your clothes, you're throwing out your entire cleansing process and bringing in gazillions of little bacteria from your old clothes onto your newly washed and exfoliated body. I can promise you the odor will run rampant.

- You don't have to iron if you don't want to, you don't have to use a fabric softener is you don't want to, but whether you want to or not, if you want to stay sweet-smelling, and not sweat-smelling then wash your clothes, and along with that wear a new change of clothes every time, or even every other time you shower. Trust me, it helps.

Trim excess hair

- If you tend to sweat excessively under your arms, then trimming or shaving your underarm hair can help you to stay odor free.

- The longer the underarm hair then the more likely it will be that you will begin to give off a stench when you start sweating.

- Bacteria have a better chance of thriving when there is more hair. And even regular washing will have trouble in dislodging or keeping those little germs away from your pits.

Dry out thoroughly

- Whenever possible either use a blow dryer to thoroughly dry out problem areas, or if you have the time allow yourself to dry out under a fan (this works!).

- You will still be slightly damp no matter how hard your dry yourself. This can mean the deodorant you're applying is not quite as effective. The best thing is if you can take the time out to dry yourself thoroughly.

Water

Water is the most natural resource on the face of this earth, one of the most necessary components for our survival, and we have to force ourselves to drink it because we need it.

This is why I have brought myself to the point where I prefer water over carbonated or artificial drinks.

Water is an absolute must, if you're going to fight odor and sweat, and no matter how you go about it, you will need to get some into you on a daily basis, and more than the forced down glass or two.

You will need to take in at least 6-8 glasses of water a day. That means that you can't fudge by using a small 4oz glass.

It might seem difficult right now, when you think of the tastelessness and colorlessness of water (I'm joking of course - water tastes great to my mind), but if you get yourself into a routine, it does become easier.

Recommendations:

1. One glass sometime during your morning routine,

2. One glass when you get to work, or at midmorning,

3. One glass at lunch time,

4. One glass during your mid afternoon tea break (see, that's four glasses already!)

5. One glass when you get back home

6. One glass with dinner, (if you're not eating at the time you get back home)

7. And one glass before you go to bed, or half-an-hour before you go to bed

- Go for it throughout the entire day, and don't try to cram it all in one half hour period!

- Try to squeeze in another glass of water or two when you're not looking, and let go of your carbonated beverages, you will definitely be on the right track.

- The one time that you definitely want to go above and beyond the eight glasses of water a day is when you're doing something that is labor intensive like exercising, or gardening, or playing sports, or something along those lines. At these times you will find that you sweat unconditionally, and that you need to replenish your depleted water reserves.

- If you have fever, you will more than likely sweat like a pig, so you will need to be careful about not dehydrating when you're down with the fever.

Tip: Stay hydrated, keep ice chips by your bedside to suck on, or keep a sippy cup of water by your bedside. Whatever you do, don't forget the water. It's important.

Proper Diet

Ideally your diet needs to be one that promotes proper digestion and elimination of waste products from your body. This would normally include fibrous foods as well as foods rich in vitamins and minerals.

All the junk food we grew up eating when we were kids just doesn't make the cut. To make a proper dietary change you will need to cut these foods from your menu altogether, but let's be honest here, it's not that easy.

In the beginning we really won't be able to cut out each and every single one of your favorite foods just because they're bad for us. I don't think that's a news flash for any of us.

You've known for some time now that fast- and processed- foods are bad for you, but you still haven't changed your eating habits so that means that even now, when you really need to, it will take some time for you to make this change.

Don't expect miracles. Do it gradually, and expect to see results from this only a few months later along the road. Until then, know your weaknesses where food is concerned, and duly make allowance for that.

- If you crave your chocolates, then have them by all means, but in small manageable doses. If you need your morning hit of fried bacon and hash browns then have it, but not every day.

- Cut back on the greasy burger and fries for lunch; eat a smaller bag of chips for your snack; cut down on the gallon of ice cream you go through in three days. Make these small changes, gradually and over a period of time, and you can expect to see the big changes as you go on.

- While you're making compromises with your cravings, you can include in your diet the foods which you need to keep

you healthy, and which you need to aid
you in living a sweat-free life.

Tip: To make it slightly easier for you, I have
included a list of some of the foods which you
should eat to promote a healthy sweat free life,
and some of the foods you shouldn't go near.

At the end of this particular section I have also
listed a few vitamins and minerals which you
should include in your diet, either in
supplemental pill or tablet form, or through your
daily intake of fruits, vegetables and meats.

Foods you need

You will see that this list I'm outlining in this
section isn't too specific, like for instance the very
first item I have listed is, "Foods rich in zinc". I
felt that this said it all, really. What I was trying
to get you to do with this was to look into having
are foods rich in zinc, and not the specific food
itself.

Sometimes, the very foods that I have listed as good for you might also belong to one of these overall groups, but I have listed them specifically because they serve the purpose you need very well, and serve to illustrate what type of foods I am talking about in general.

- Foods rich in zinc
- Sage
- Foods rich in chlorophyll
- Leafy greens
- Raw vegetables and fruits
- Parsley
- Broccoli
- Sprouts (good source of chlorophyll)
- Whole grains to aid in digestion
- Alfalfa
- Watermelon to cool the body
- Low fat or skimmed milk
- Calcium rich foods
- Parsley
- Lastly you should learn to cook using mono- or poly-unsaturated fats

Foods to Avoid

- Garlic
- Onions
- Fish
- Red meats
- Curries
- Strong, hot or spicy foods
- Fried foods
- Heavily sweetened foods
- Coffee
- Large amounts of black Tea
- Caffeinated beverages
- Cinnamon
- Reduce salt intake
- Avoid polysaturated fats to cook with

Vitamins and Supplements

- Zinc

- Magnesium
- Chlorophyll
- Vitamin B complex
- Calcium

Alcohol, Coffee, and Smoking

All I can say is NO.

There is absolutely no way that I can convince myself that these are good for me, and there is absolutely no way that you can make these good for you either. The bottom line is that all these three things are definitely not good for you. In fact they are downright bad for you.

They can be addictive and you can't give them up very easily, but they're not good for you. And maybe the most innocuous one among the three that I have mentioned in the heading, is coffee.

- Millions of people guzzle this down as if it were their salvation to staying alive and wired, (and maybe it is!), but that still doesn't make it good for you, nor does it make an essential dietary item.

- Being "alive and wired" is definitely not how you want your metabolism to be if you're prone to sweating.

- You might not be wired by drinking in moderation, or smoking, but the smell of both can linger in your body for hours causing your perspiration to smell.

- Not only that it can also remain on your hair and your clothing until such time as you can find it within you to wash it off. But going back to the wired part, if you sweat excessively or if you know that sweat when you have alcohol, either stay away from it in it's entirety of only take it in moderation.

- Too much alcohol, besides giving you a hangover, can also make your system "wired", and this will almost definitely bring out the sweating maniac in you.

So, coffee bad, alcohol bad, and smoking bad. All I can say is have fun in trying to give these up. These are three of the hardest things to give up, and along with trying to actually get some water into your system, these can contribute towards the most trying times for you. Persevere though and you will be amply rewarded.

Clothing

This is an important section since clothing plays an important role in our daily lives. Besides having to launder your clothing on a regular basis, and change out of it on a regular basis as well, it does help if you are armed with the right type of clothes to wear when fighting sweat.

- If you live in a hot climate then silks are definitely not on the cards for you, unless you step out of an air conditioned house, to an air conditioned car, to an air conditioned office, and don't do anything more strenuous than lifting a pen.

- Silks look good, feels good, and they also show every single sweat mark that you have. They can also be sweat inducing for some people. If you're in this category, then stay away from silk.

Some people, such as me, are affected by this even when they're in cold climates, and will find that silk just isn't on the cards for them. In fact some people find themselves sweating even when it is freezing outside. This can actually be attributed to the effect of bundling up warmly.

You would like to stay warm, but sometimes you can overkill and dress so warmly that you feel like you're in the middle summer! I know so because I am one of those people.
As mentioned before, I dress in layers. You can take off the layers according to the temperature and you won't be stuck with just one type of clothing that is making you feel uncomfortable.

Tip: Wear a thick winter coat which you can take off anytime, a thinner undercoat which you can wear in all but the most freezing of conditions, and your normal clothes which are mostly the same type of clothes you wear during summer.

Below is a small list of the clothing you should and shouldn't wear. These also include different types of clothing as well:

What to wear and what not to wear

- Wear cottons, linen, silks, and wool -- all natural fiber clothing.

- Don't wear artificial fiber clothing -- these are absolutely the worst type of clothes that you can wear when you have a perspiration problem.

- Wear light colored clothing -- whites and pastels work best in these situations

- Don't wear dark clothing -- stay away from black and dark colored clothing, they will attract and trap heat.

- Wear loose fitting clothes -- you should have a free flow of air going through your clothes so that your skin can breathe

- Don't wear clingy, tight clothing -- no air flow if you wear these, need I say more?

- Avoid high necked clothing like turtlenecks. They can give rise to more sweat problems than you're willing to deal with!

Some Natural deodorants

Here we are at the natural deodorants. Below are a few natural deodorants which can be used to help combat perspiration and odor from sweating. I have also listed a few of the ingredients which you can find in commercially marketed natural deodorants.

These are over and above the ones that you can create yourself, or that you can buy in specialty stores.

Some ingredients which you can expect to find in natural deodorants.

- Antibacterial, anti-inflammatory and deodorizing essential oils such as Tea Tree, Sage, Citrus oils, Witch Hazel and Rosemary among others.
- Aloe Vera
- Vitamin E
- Lichen
- Seaweed
- Purified Clay
- Stearic Acid -- non toxic chemical ingredient
- Sodium Stearate -- non toxic chemical ingredient

- Allantoin -- non toxic chemical ingredient

Ingredients to avoid:

- Aluminum Salts -- prevents sweat by clogging the pores
- Boric Acid
- Butylated Hydroxytoluene (BHT) -- is a preservative and a suspected carcinogen
- Triclosan -- is a synthetic antibacterial
- Propylene glycol -- has been known to cause an accumulation of lactic acid waste in body cells
- Methyl paraben
- Sorbitan monostearate
- Petrolatum or petroleum jelly
- Dibutyl phthalate (DBP)
- Fragrance (Parfum) -- the fragrance used is mainly chemical based
- Talc -- this is used as a filler, and reduces overall moisture

Ammonium Alum or Potassium Alum

You can find this as a crystallized stick, and this is one of the most natural deodorants out there. It is not expensive and has a long shelf life (about a year so) you can be certain that you will be getting value for money.

This is however not an antiperspirant so you will still sweat. It is a very good antibacterial agent which cuts down on the bacteria buildup which in turn reduces odor.

This is a natural deodorant that is gaining in popularity as word about it spreads. A few years ago many people would have given you a blank stare if you went and asked for an ammonium alum deodorant. These days the tide is turning for natural deodorants and ammonium alum is going straight to the top of many people's lists.

This is also my most favored method of dealing with sweat, seconded only by the use of essential oils.

Baking Soda

Baking soda works to neutralize any odors and kills odor producing bacteria, which is also the reason why our mothers used to keep an open package of baking soda in the fridge!

If you prefer something that is ready made, you can look for a natural deodorant which contains baking soda. But be warned that these deodorants may also contain other substances which aren't as good for you. Check out the list of "bad" ingredients which you might find at the very beginning of this section.

If you want to use baking soda *au natural* then all you need to do is to dust a little bit of it over the problematic areas. Cornstarches also work along the same principles and can be dusted on you in lieu of baking soda if you've run out (although you might feel odd at first, dusting yourself with cornstarch, it can and does work).

On the other hand you can use a mixture of baking soda and cornstarch to deal with your sweat problems. Just take equal parts baking soda and cornstarch and apply.

Herbal tea deodorant

Antibacterial herbs: peppermint, sage, or coriander.

- When it is cool, dilute it with mineral water, add a few drops of your favorite essential oil, and apply on your underarms, and other sweat prone areas for cooling freshness.

- Make sure that you're dry before you put on your clothes, otherwise this method will just be useless. Bacteria thrive in damp dark places and your underarms will present just such an opportunity for them to thrive if you dress in a hurry without drying.

Find more tea in the herbal teas section.

To make your basic easy herbal tea:

1. Take 1 teaspoon of whatever dried herb you're using, or 3 teaspoons of the fresh version of the herb.
2. Pour 1 cup of boiling water over it, and allow it to steep for about 5-10 minutes, before straining it.

Tip: What's tricky is knowing when enough time has passed for the steeping process. Some herbs require less time than others, and if you're going to be drinking the tea, then it becomes a matter of personal preference as to how strong you want your tea to be.

Body Powders (Talc)

Baby powders, or normal body powders which you can use to combat the effects of sweating. These are best used after a shower, and after you have dried off completely.

- Apply a light dusting of the powder of your choice onto your armpits, and anywhere else that you might sweat (or all over your body).

It gives you a refreshing feel and can keep you feeling fresh for some time to come.

Essential Oils

Essential oils are used for relaxation, or simply a luxuriating bath, you can use any of the essential oils listed below. They also have the added benefit of fighting odors.

Bath:

- Add a few drops of the essential oil into your bath. To get a better bath experience you can learn to mix and match the scents that suit you best so that you don't end up smelling like a hothouse flower when all you wanted was a clean mountain-fresh scent.

Tip: You should also note that some essential oils are not to be used if you are pregnant, breast feeding, or expecting to become pregnant. Also, if you are on medications of any sort, or you have a health condition, consult with your physician before you start using any of the essential oils.

Essential oils:

- Orange -- antibacterial
- Sandalwood -- antibacterial

- Bergamot -- antiseptic, deodorant
- Peppermint - antiseptic
- Cypress -- antiseptic, deodorant
- Jasmine -- antibacterial
- Rose -- antibacterial
- Rosemary (avoid if pregnant) -- antiseptic
- Lavender -- antibacterial, deodorant
- Myrrh -- antibacterial
- Juniper berry -- antiseptic
- Oak bark -- antibacterial
- Sage -- antibacterial (avoid if pregnant)
- Thyme -- antibacterial
- Orange Blossom -- antibacterial
- Lemon -- antibacterial
- Patchouli -- antiseptic, deodorant
- Petitgrain -- deodorant
- Calendula -- antibacterial
- Neroli -- antiseptic, deodorant
- Lime -- antibacterial
- Ginger -- antibacterial
- Witch Hazel -- anti-inflammatory, astringent

- Rosewood -- antiseptic, deodorant

- Chamomile (avoid if pregnant) -- antiseptic

- Clary Sage -- antibacterial, deodorant

- Eucalyptus -- antiseptic, deodorant

Tip: The few last essential oils which I've mentioned above might be too pungent to use by itself for some people. I have a sensitive nose and prefer to mix these oils to create a more pleasing mixture. If you can't stand the smell of these, or even like the smell, then I would suggest that you mix and match these oils.

- Tea tree (mixed with something else) -- antibacterial

- Margosa -- antibacterial

- Neem -- antibacterial

- Coriander -- anti-inflammatory, deodorant

You can also use these essential in the shower by adding a few drops to a washcloth or your favorite shower gel.

Tip: Apply a few drops to a washcloth and apply the oil (mixture in most cases and depending upon my mood), under my arms especially, around my neck and just about everywhere else!

Citrus Wash

You will need:

- The juice of 1 Lemon, freshly squeezed
- 10 drops Lemon essential oil
- 2 oz. Water

Steps:

- Mix the ingredients well together.

To use:

- Wipe sweat prone areas (excepting the genital area), with this citrus wash. Especially wipe the underarms thoroughly with this wash using either your hands or a washcloth.

- The remainder of the citrus wash that you didn't use can be placed in the fridge,

preferably in a darkened glass airtight
container, and used for about 1-2 days.

Tip: This citrus wash is always best used when
prepared fresh, so don't prepare a lot of it and
keep it on hand. All you really need are the basic
ingredients to hand, and the time it takes to
squeeze a lemon.

Lavender Water

You will need:

- 5 drops Lavender oil
- 2 cups distilled Water

Steps:

- Mix the lavender oil and the distilled
  water together, and pour into a dark glass
  bottle preferably, although a normal glass
  bottle will also work fine.

- Make sure the bottle is airtight.

To use:

- Dab the lavender solution onto the areas which perspire the most.

- To carry it around with you, simply pour some of the mixture into a smaller bottle.

Tip: Store the rest out of direct sunlight. I have found that periodically applying this can be helpful in keeping you feeling fresh throughout the day.

Lavender and Thyme Wash

You will need:

- 5 drops Thyme oil
- 5 drops Lavender oil

Steps:

- Add the thyme and the lavender to your bath.

- Alternately you can add it to your shower gel, or barring that add it to a washcloth and rub yourself with it.

- If you are using the washcloth method, make sure that you dilute the oil by first wetting the washcloth.

Herbs

The herbs listed below are good by themselves or mixed with other herbs mentioned. Keep in mind that there are only a few types of herbs that actually reduce sweating are not as numerous as those that can induce sweating!

Also keep in mind that I haven't given you any specific directions on what to do with any of the herbs, except in the "Herbal teas" section, for the very simple reason that I am not a qualified herbalist.

I am in no position to tell you what amounts of the herbs you should take.
Sweating is such a personal thing, the herbs needed for you will not necessarily be the same herbs, or the amounts which I myself am using. Different people need/react differently too.

This is why your best course of action would be to consult with a trained and qualified herbalist to find the right dosages and the right herbs for you.

As for the tea recipes which I have given you in the next section, these are the standard tea recipes and can be drunk by just about anyone. However, if you are pregnant, or taking any kind of medication, you will first want to consult your doctor to see whether these teas are good for you. Below is the list of herbs.

- Sage -- since sage is such an all rounder when it comes to sweating and preventing or minimizing it, I have dedicated a separate section all by itself to sage, which comes after the "Herbal Teas" section.

- Astragalus -- reduces sweating, balances the body's sweat actions appropriately

- Nettle -- provides relief for your body from overheating

- Hops -- soothes

- Peppermint -- gives your body a cooling effect

- Milk Thistle -- improves the functioning of the liver

- White Peony Root -- aids in the loss of sweating, balances your body

- Oats -- relieve stress if you are sweating due to stress or anxiety

- Fennel -- aids liver function

- Motherwort -- relaxes and soothes

- Sarsaparilla -- good for hot flashes

- Licorice Root -- good for hot flashes

- Red Raspberry -- good for hot flashes, also cools the body

Herbal teas

Here are a few of herbal teas for you to get started with. The remedies I give you here are for informational purposes only.

Once again, I would strongly recommend that if you are pregnant, breast feeding, taking medication of any sort or have a health problem, consult with your doctor first, and/ or a trained herbalist. Being safe is the best way to go.

These professionals can better guide you along the right path, and help you to choose the herbs which are best suited for you. Remember, I'm not a qualified medical practitioner or herbalist.

They can also inform you on how long and how often you can take each of these safely, please confer with a trained herbalist. They can tell you which herbs can be taken on a daily basis, and which herbs can only be taken for a certain time frame only.

Raspberry tea

Drinking raspberry tea will help to produce a natural cooling effect on your system.

You will need:

- 1-2 tsp dried Raspberry leaf
- 1 cup Water
- Honey to taste

Steps:

- Boil the water first. Place the dried raspberry leaf in a suitable container and pour the boiling water over the leaves.

- Cover the teapot and allow the tea to stand for 8-10 minutes, then strain, and add honey to taste before drinking.

- This tea can be drunk about once or twice a day.

Peppermint tea

Drinking peppermint tea produces a similar cooling effect to that of drinking raspberry leaf tea.

You will need:

- 1-2 tsp dried Peppermint leaf
- 1 cup Water
- Honey to taste

Steps:

- As with the raspberry leaf tea, boil the water first. Add the dried peppermint to a teapot or a suitable mug, preferably with an infuser, and pour the water over the peppermint.

- Steep the tea for 8-10 minutes, keeping the teapot covered so that the potency of the tea isn't diminished. Add honey only if you want it.

- Not everyone likes honey with their peppermint tea, so you will need to taste it beforehand to decide whether you want to honey.

Nettle tea

Nettle tea can provide relief from overheating. You can have about 3 cups of tea a day. Powdered nettle can also be added to smoothies if you don't want to have the tea. Just use one or two teaspoons per glass.

You will need:

- 3 tsp of fresh Nettle leaves (or 1tsp dried nettle)
- 1 cup Water
- Honey to taste

Steps:

- Add the water and the nettle leaves to a suitable container and boil for about 2-4 minutes. Take off the stove and strain.

- Add honey to taste and drink.

Astragalus tea

You can drink this tea about once or twice a day.

You will need:

- 3 tbsp of dried Astragalus
- 3 cups of Water

Steps:

- You will need to take a suitable pot, enamel is better if you have it. Place the water and the dried Astragalus in the pot and set on the fire.

- Bring the water to a boil and simmer for about 20 minutes. Strain and cool the tea before serving.

Motherwort tea

Motherwort taken daily should be limited to two cups a day. You can use either the leaves, flowers or the stem of Motherwort when using as an herbal tea.

You will need:

- 2 tsp of dried Motherwort
- 1 cup boiling water

Steps:

- First boil the water. Add the motherwort to a teapot and pour the boiling water over it. Cover and steep for about 7-10 minutes. Strain, and then drink, adding honey if necessary.

Fennel Tea

Fennel aids in the proper functioning of the liver, which in turn can help you to stay healthy. This is also a great tea to be drunk after meals as it also aids in digestion.

You will need:

- 1-1½ tsp ground Fennel seeds
- 1 cup Water

Steps:

- Boil the water first, add the ground fennel to a mug or a teapot, and pour the boiling over it. Allow this to steep for about 5-7 minutes or until desired strength is achieved.

Lemonbalm and Fennel Tea

This is a nice combination of herbs to use, and you can drink it about twice a day. Both the herbs have anti-bacterial properties.

You will need:

- 1 tsp ground Fennel seeds
- 1 tsp crushed Lemonbalm
- 1½ cups water

Steps:

- Boil the water first. Place the fennel and the lemonbalm in a teapot, and pour the boiling water over them.

- Steep for about 10 minutes, strain, and then drink. Add honey only if you feel you need it.

Oatstraw tea

This is great stress relieving tea and can help to calm you down, and is just as good as taking oats. This in turn can help to bring down your metabolism which can help to control your sweating.

You will need:

- 1-1½ tsp dried Oatstraw
- 1 cup Water

Steps:

- Bring the water to a boil first. Place the oatstraw in a tea pot and pour the boiling water over it. Allow it to steep for about 8-10 minutes before drinking it.

- If you desire a stringer tea, add more oatstraw but leave the steeping time of the tea between 8-10 minutes.

Stress reliever tea

A combination of Peppermint, Lemonbalm and Fennel made into a tea and taken just before going to bed can reduce stress or anxiety. This in turn can stop anxiety or stress induced sweating.

You will need:

- 5 tsp of dried Peppermint
- 5 tsp of dried Lemonbalm
- 5 tsp of ground Fennel seeds
- 1 cup Water

Steps:

- You will first need to mix all of the dried herbs together. Since this will produce more tea mixture than necessary, you can store it in an airtight container for further use.

- Bring the water to a boil. Place 1 tsp of the peppermint, lemonbalm and fennel mixture into a teapot and pour the boiling water over it.

- Steep this, covered, for about 7-10 minutes, or until you achieve a desired strength, then strain and drink. If needed add honey to taste and/ or lemon.

Sweat relieving tea

This is a great tasting tea and can be drunk at any time of day.

You will need:

- 3 tsp fresh Sage leaves (dried will also do)
- 1tsp of dried stinging Nettle
- 1tsp of dried Hops
- 1 tsp of fresh Strawberry leaves (dried will also do)
- 1 tsp of fresh Walnut leaves
- 1 tsp of fresh Rose petals
- 4 cups of Water

Steps:

- Place the water in a suitable saucepan, enamel is best, and bring to a boil. Add the herbs into the boiling water and cover the pan.

- Remove from the heat almost immediately and set aside to steep for

about one hour. Strain the tea, add honey
to taste if you need it.

Sage

Sage is an herb and it is separately written here in
all my many efforts at finding a proper natural
remedy to help me combat my sweaty problems,
I found that sage was one of the better
recommended herbs to do so.

Personally speaking I didn't find that sage alone
worked wonders for me, I had to also make
certain lifestyle changes as well. To that extent I
decided that sage, over and above the other herbs,
deserved a section all of its own away from the
other herbs.

It's a love it or hate it thing with sage. Some
people love the taste of sage and some people just
can't stand it. There are of course others that
would try anything that can help their sweating
problems even if they don't like the taste of the
sage.

There is also the theory that to help you combat sweating, sage tea needs to be drunk cold to stop sweating, otherwise if it is drunk while still hot, it can induce sweating.

It has also been said that when you drink sage tea, that the effects can be seen for up to about two hours. In other words, you can stay sweat free for about two hours or so after drinking a cooling cup of sage tea.

*Note: If you are pregnant, or expecting to become pregnant avoid sage in all of its forms. If you suffer from epilepsy, sage can cause epileptic strokes.

Sage Tea

This is the more normally used version of the sage tea, and can be drunk either hot or cold.

You will need:

- 1 tbsp fresh Sage leaves
- 1 cup of Water
- 1 Lemon wedge
- Honey to taste

Steps:

- First you will need to boil the water. When this is done, take the water off the heat and add the sage leaves. Leave it to steep for about 5-8 minutes, no more as it can turn out too strong.

- Strain the tea into a cup after the allotted time, (5 minutes for a lighter strength tea, and 8 minutes for a stronger tasting tea). Squeeze in the lemon and add the honey to taste.

- To drink it cold, it is best left to cool and then poured over ice. If you want (if you don't like ice), you can even cool it in the refrigerator.

You can also find sage teabags without having to go to all the trouble of using fresh sage. Sage teabags can be found in health food stores, or barring that, you can even find it in online health food stores or suppliers.

Prepare the prepackaged sage teabags according to instructions on the packaging.

Sage and Rhubarb Iced Tea

It sounds absolutely disgusting, but I have to say that it is quite nice when all is said and done.

Note: preparing this can be a little messy.

You will need:

- 2-4 tbsp fresh Sage leaves or blossoms
- 1 cup Rhubarb, chopped
- ½ cup fresh tart Red Cherries, pitted (the canned or the frozen variety will also do)
- 2 Teabags (the normal variety)
- ¼ cup Honey, (or to taste)
- ½ tbsp Balsamic Vinegar
- Lemon slices for Garnish
- 3 cups Water

Steps:

- Take a saucepan and place ½ cup of water, the cherries and the rhubarb inside, and place on the fire. You will need to bring it to a boil, the cover and leave to simmer on a low heat for about 30 minutes.

- When this is done, take a large sieve and strain the rhubarb and cherry mixture through it, mashing the cooked fruit in the process to get the most out of it. You can use a spoon to mash and strain the fruit.

- You will then need to place the strained fruit mixture in the saucepan you used earlier (discarding the strained pulp in the sieve).

- Bring the cherry and rhubarb mixture to a boil and add the sage, the teabags and the balsamic vinegar. Take it off the fire immediately and leave somewhere to steep for about 5-8 minutes.

- You will then need to strain the mixture again, this time taking out the fresh sage and the teabags. This is your sage tea concentrate.

- To make the iced tea, you will need to let the tea concentrate cool for a little while. Then, taking a suitable pitcher, you will need to add the remaining water ($2\frac{1}{2}$ cups) and the tea mixture.

- Stir well, adding the honey (mostly to taste, so add more, or less depending on what you want).

- Also, liquid honey works best for this recipe as the solidified honey takes longer to dissolve in the colder water than it does in hot water.

- Add the lemon slices for garnishing and either serve on ice, or add the ice to the pitcher itself.

Tip: Another thing that I like to do is to add a little lemon juice as well just before serving the tea. You can experiment with this and see what mixtures and quantities you like.

Tip: It also makes a great party tea for those long hot days of summer with its vibrant red color and the added effect the sage has of reducing sweat.

Sage and Tomato

Blend about 2 tsp of Sage with a glass of tomato juice to have a sweat reducing drink.

Sage Tea Wash

- Use the Sage Tea recipe which I mentioned earlier, but leave out the honey if you don't feel comfortable with it. Otherwise use the tea as-is, only leaving it to cool.

- You can use it as a great body wash to help stop, or more to the point, reduce your sweating. For people with hyperhidrosis this is also another viable method they can look into for treating their problem.

Sage Tinctures and Essential Oil

Essential oil needs to be diluted with carrier oil such as almond oil, jojoba oil, wheat germ oil, or any other such appropriate oil. Both the tincture and the oils can be used in the same manner, by applying to the problem areas.

You will however need to keep away from the sensitive genital areas, as well as the face.

And as I mentioned earlier sage should *not* be taken by pregnant women, or women expecting to become pregnant.

The Unusuals

This section contains a collection of odds and ends you can use in your fight against odor and sweat. They are mainly home remedies and you should take them as such. I only included them because they do work, if only you go about it with an open mind.

- If you have a sweat, or heat, rash try bathing the affected areas with strongly brewed black tea everyday (no sugar please!).

- For sweaty hands, soak them in a plate of strongly brewed, cooled, black tea for about 2-4 minutes. Be aware that your hands could take on a brownish color if left to soak too long!

- For smelly feet, soak them in hot, not boiling, black tea for about 20 minutes.

- Chew on parsley leaves to cut out sweat induced odor.

- Take a wheat grass pill (500mg) to combat sweat odor.

- Grate, juice and strain a turnip, and rub the juice of it on dry underarms to stop sweating.

- Juice a dozen radishes, mix with ¼ teaspoon of glycerin and use as a foot deodorant, this is best used before going to bed.

- Take 2 teaspoons of Apple Cider Vinegar along with 2 teaspoons of Honey on an empty stomach to reduce sweating.

- Use a tomato and sage mixture diluted with water, as a wash for sweat affected areas. This is great to get rid of odor.

Homeopathy

Homeopathy has worked for me with dealing with my sweating I have listed below a few homeopathic remedies which can be good for you. Homeopathy is best left to the experts in my opinion, so I have not given any dosage instructions.

For detailed instructions on dosages and which remedy us the best for your type sweating, please consult a homeopathic physician.

I have given first the treatment, and following that the symptoms that pertain to that particular treatment. It goes along the general lines of, if your symptoms are so and so, this treatment is the one for you.

- Acidum hydrofluoricum -- if your sweat smells offensive; if cold weather relieves your sweating; if walking relieves your sweating; and if the sweat is worse on your head and scalp area.

- Calcarea carbonica -- if your skin is damp or clammy; if it tends to become worse in wet weather, or from exertion or mental and emotional stimuli; if there is s sour smell emanating; if you are sensitive to colder weather and you are also overweight.

- Lycopodium -- if your sweat smells unpleasant; if the perspiration is concentrated more on the feet and the arms.

- Graphites -- if you have worse symptoms during the night time; if you are stout or overweight; and if your perspiration is offensive or foul smelling.

- Psorinum -- if odor is constant and persists even after washing; if the skin looks dull or dirty.

- Kali phosphorica -- if you sweat early in the morning; if cold weather affects you; if mental stimuli such as stress and anxiety affects you adversely.

- Silicea -- if your sweat smells offensive; if you sweat mostly on the feet or underarms; and if you tend to have chilly hands or feet.

Deodorants and Breast Cancer

There are many speculations about deodorants and breast cancer. Many studies are still being conducted on this subject.

I'm sure that the truth will be found sometime in the future, but until then there can only be speculation. And speculation is most definitely a two way street!

Personally, I prefer to sit back and watch the developments unfold. Obviously somebody has to be right, or both sides have to be partially correct. Until such time as any result can be verified as being the truth, I prefer to err on the side of caution.

There is a possibility that there could be absolutely no connection between the two, but then again so could the conspiracy theorists be right, and deodorants could be one of the leading causes of breast cancer (and other diseases too!).

The best thing to do in this case is to be aware of the facts. Take as many precautions as you can, but not be too paranoid that it interferes with your life. It's useless avoiding deodorants and other such "bad" things only to live a hermit-like existence!

Here are some of the facts at hand to make up our own minds, and our own decisions:

- There is no conclusive link between breast cancer and deodorants.

- Studies have been conducted to this end. At this time the results depend greatly on how you view the entire situation.

- Tests conducted on breast cancer tumors have shown that substances to be found in deodorants, and which do not naturally occur in the body, are found in the tumors as well, leaving the field wide open to speculation.

- There is also the popularly held belief that by shaving your underarms, you're giving the chemicals in the deodorants the ability to more freely get into our systems.

- On the converse side, it is argued that the lymphatic system would stop any type of alien substance from entering our bodies therefore it would not be possible for deodorants to lead to breast cancer or indeed, any other disease.

- It is also said that the ingredients used in deodorants are not easily absorbed into the skin and only act on very superficial level.

Both sides are practical and both sides make a good case. The problem here lies in not what the evidence suggests but how much we are willing to go along with the evidence.

To that end, your own life's experiences as well as our belief system is the one thing that will make the ultimate decision for us. How can I say that, right? If something has been proven beyond all shadow of a doubt to be bad for you, that it could cause irreparable harm to you, why would you continue on that same self destructive tack?

If I may, I will take a very straightforward example that illustrates this very clearly, and which is still prevalent in our societies today. What am I talking about? Smoking.

It has been proven to cause lung cancer, there is a warning on the front of each packet of cigarettes, and yet there are still millions, even billions of people in the world today who smoke at least one or two cigarettes a day, if not a pack.

You will naturally enough and in due course make up your own mind, and not because someone pressures you to do so, but because you interpret the facts you're given in a certain way. This is natural, and this is human nature.

What you need to do now, is to decide whether you want to continue using chemical based antiperspirants and deodorants, or whether you want to try natural deodorants and methods for preventing or dealing with sweat.

But since you're reading this book which means that you are looking natural deodorants and other natural sweat and odor prevention methods, we can say that you're headed in that direction anyway.

On my part, I have to say, (and just in case you haven't already guessed!), that I prefer to use more natural methods.

This is not only because I started getting adverse reactions to many deodorants and antiperspirants that I have used, but also because with age, I am becoming more careful and picky about what I put in and on my body.

In the Natural Course of Events

Since natural is the game of the day, it is now in the natural course of events, time for me to take my leave of you. Hopefully everything that you have read in this book has enlightened you on the topic of sweat, and hopefully you will have found it to be of assistance to you.

A few things to remember:

- Using the proper natural methods which are suitable for you, you can control your sweating

- If at any point in time you feel that you might be sweating overly much or not at all, then consult your doctor.

- And most of all, it's alright to sweat, it's a natural part of life to do so. Just remember to follow the few simple guidelines laid out in the book and you should be alright.

The rest as they say, is history. You will now be able to stand tall and walk proud anywhere you go. They key thing here is to be confident within yourself, and to put your best, well ventilated, foot forward.